HOW TO SELL PERSONAL TRAINNG

How To Build Your Personal Training Clientele and Business Faster and Easier Than You Ever Thought Possible

www.thefiture.co

EMAIL ME AT GREG@FITURE.CO

Section 1- Sales

"If you can master sales you can write your own check"

Personal training is definitely a business that has grown over the years and it is a profession that is extremely fun and satisfying. I believe most personal trainers get in the business of personal training because they want to help people and the idea of using fitness as a vehicle is very attractive to them.

Personal trainers are attracted to energy and the environment of the gym and when they know that they can truly change someone's life while making a living then most personal trainers are sold and want to know how to get started. When a personal trainer begins their certification process they study the human body, how to perform the exercises correctly, and how to do specific tests on clients to make sure they are safe and getting results.

Once a personal trainer gets certified they then look for a gym or studio to start training people. This is where it gets tricky and confusing for most personal trainers because they soon find out that clients are not knocking their doors down to have them train them.

In fact, the personal trainer usually finds out that the act of getting clients is intimidating and frustrating because that is the one thing the certification and education system did not teach them….how to sell and market yourself as a personal trainer.

In this book I am going to show you a system for solving your problem and giving you the control to have as many clients as you want as long as you master these principles.

This system has worked for many of the trainers I have mentored and coached and it will work for you.

In selling and marketing yourself as a trainer you want to make sure that you have fun and you know specific things like how to position yourself, how to emotionally sell, what your sales mentality is , and most important how to get clients in front of you so you can sell them.

Let's get started with mindset.

Your Mindset

In order to sell personal training you must first believe that everyone can use the help of a personal trainer. Think about most athletes and what level of athleticism and workout experience they have and also how they invest in having a personal trainer to help them reach their highest potential. Anyone can benefit from a personal trainer or coach because we all know that when we have someone who is watching over us and pushing us we tend to train harder and focus better.

Most personal trainers get the right credentials and have their heart in the right place as far as wanting to help people change their lives but they usually have a hard time selling their services because they have a hang up with money and associating asking people to pay them for their knowledge and expertise as being greedy or even worse they are afraid of being considered a "salesman".

There is nothing wrong for trading your value and expertise in fitness, which you worked extremely hard for and paid good money to get certified, for money. I need you to think about several reasons why people hire personal trainers and write them down because in order to sell the personal trainer experience you must sell yourself.

Some of the reasons why I believe and teach other trainers on why people hire us is for the following
- accountability
- motivation
- knowledge on how to put their exercises together
- a friend or therapist to help them with their life

Now there are plenty more for why people hire a personal trainer but these are some common ones. The next thing you want to do is accept your sales role.

Accepting your Sales Role

Most people have a very negative opinion or belief about sales and what selling actually means. The first thing you must do is accept that you are selling to help and that you DO NOT need to turn into some other personality in order to sell personal training. The mistake trainers make is they believe that they are not enough of a personality to sell people on their training so they try to morph into some "salesman" that they have seen on TV or experienced and when you try to be something you are not, you will struggle mightily to sell because the client will be able to pick up on that.

When you decide that you are going to be proud to sell your packages and yourself then you will see a significant increase in your sales effectiveness. You will have more excitement and you will communicate better because you will be congruent with what you are doing. If you are not comfortable with the idea of selling then it will show and it will take longer to be successful because there will be something holding you back.

Reframe how you look at what selling is. All selling is, is the activity of finding clients who have a problem that you can solve and communicating clearly to them that you have the answer to their problem. You are actually doing the client a disservice if you don't sell them what you have to offer.

Personal training is your way of contributing to society's problem of being overweight, unhappy, and insecure with themselves. Be proud to be a personal trainer and what you are offering. A common problem is most trainers start off with little money so they have a tendency to sell with the poverty syndrome. Read below to learn more about this.

Poverty Syndrome or Selling out of your own Pocket

A common mistake many personal trainers make when they are trying to sell their packages are they either automatically assume that they are overpriced or they sell the package that they (the personal trainer not client) can afford.

An example would be if you are a personal trainer who just got out of college and have never paid your own bills before or currently your bank account is not where you would like it to be then you may think a $100 or $200 per month may be too expensive because it is expensive to you.

Avoid this mindset like the plague because if you sell from this standpoint you are going to have an extremely hard time selling your programs to your potential clients because they will feel that intuitive feeling that you do not believe in your product or you might be overcharging.

People can sense when you feel uneasy, and naturally, if you feel uneasy then they will feel uneasy and it makes it incredibly hard to sell anything because there will be that feeling that just seems like it is not right.

The best way to fix your mindset when it comes to poverty syndrome or selling out of your pocket is to actually practice for asking for an extremely large sum of money over and over again to get used to just saying it and realizing that money is just money and other people may be in a great place financially and cannot wait to hire a personal trainer who can speed up their results.

Many clients value having someone tell them what to do and giving someone else control of what their workout program should be so essentially they are paying for workout and time efficiency. This is very valuable to a lot of people so don't be bashful to ask them for the money. This leads to the next subject which human beings in general have a fear of and that is the fear of failing.

Fear of Failure

The reason why most trainers are afraid to sell is because they are afraid to fail and be told "no". The big mistake that is made early on is when someone tells them "no" they cannot seem to not take the "no" personally.

What I mean is when someone rejects them they take it as if the person is saying that they are a bad person. This is a big mistake that you will want to avoid because when you do this you are setting up big obstacles in the selling process such as making phone calls, sending emails, or asking for the sale.

When you are afraid of failure you will consistently find ways to not ask for the sale because you are afraid of hearing no. You will not directly ask for a yes or a no. You will not call the potential clients because they may say no to you so you make an excuse that you are "too busy "doing other things such as writing up a workout or researching things you already know so you don't have to face reality in the face that the person may say no.

But by being afraid and not even asking for what it is you want which can be the appointment, sale, or upgrade, you are forgetting that there is the very real possibility that they may say yes.

Always focus on the positive on what you and the client have to gain when you are selling. If you need some tips on how to get over the fear of failure read below.

How to get over the fear of failure

The best way to get over fear of failure which I have learned over time is by doing drills such as spending an hour per day approaching as many people as possible to hear no. The entire goal of the drill is to go out and ask people to take some form of an action and have them say no to you and once you get one no keep going until you get another one and another one.

The point of this drill is to have you hear no so many times that it thickens your skin and it proves to you that hearing no is not that bad at all. In fact, you will shock yourself with how many people will say yes to you because of you simply just asking.

This can be the greatest confidence booster because everything is about confidence and how comfortable you feel in asking for the sale. The more confident you are from asking for the sale to the presentation of information, the more likely your chances of selling more clients.

You may resist this challenge in the beginning because it is scary but if you force yourself to do it, it will be one of the best investments you will ever make because once you get over or at least learn how to manage the fear of failure you will be removing obstacles that hold you back from being more successful.

There are specific actions you can take to increase your confidence so you can feel better about the sales process and they are below.

How to build more confidence in selling yourself

The best ways to build confidence in yourself is to take control of your daily habits and what you think and do. Some things that have helped me and most definitely can help you are

- Taking care of your appearance (nice fitting clothes, nice haircut, nice athletic shoes etc.)
- reading and studying sales books by authors such as

Tom Hopkins, Brian Tracy, and Jeffrey Gitomer
- Listening to self-help podcasts that build your confidence, communication, sales skills, time management skills, leadership skills, marketing skills etc.
- going to seminars that teach you more sales, marketing, leadership, and communication skills
- network with people who are earning more money and success than you and try to pick their brain as often as possible
- surround yourself with positive people that make you feel like you can succeed and eliminate as quickly as possible the negative naysayers from your environment
- pay close attention to what kinds of foods give you energy and help you to recover
- make sure to budget out "you time" where you do fun things for yourself
- reward yourself once a week for doing a good job and reaching a goal
- always be grateful and have fun

Create goals for yourself

When you first start personal training you are going to want to make sure that you think about where you want to end up long term. There are several different things you will want to do in order to create the career and lifestyle that you want.

The first thing is what kind of schedule do you want to have? It is very tempting to think you will take anybody who wants to train at any time and work as many hours as you possibly can. The problem with that is if you don't think about how you are going to structure your days, you will end up burning yourself out because you will not have enough rest time in your day to recover and recuperate and it will cause a feeling of being stuck.

So make sure that you think through how you want your day to be structured.

The next thing you will want to do is come up with what kind of income do you want to achieve and create timelines and specific plans to reach them. What kind of income you want to make will determine how much you want to charge for your services, where you will advertise, and how you position yourself. This will also dictate how many sales presentations you will need to make in order to reach your goals.

This will help you decide how you want to communicate your sales message and put together your own customized message that is focused. A big mistake trainers make is they don't target who they want to sell and they want to sell everyone for the fear of missing out on money and they end up not creating a compelling enough message to attract the specific people they want.

This leads to deciding how you want to position yourself and how to use every way of communication in order to get your message out. The key thing here is consistency in your message. This means the way you dress, talk, advertise, sell etc is all congruent with communicating the exact message you are looking to give.

If you are serious on making a lot of personal training sales and growing your business then I highly suggest that you follow this 3 step sales process that we will be talking about in this next section.

This process has made me and many other trainers a lot of money. When you apply this method in your sales process you will significantly improve your confidence as well as your sales because it is systematic and it is my belief that anything that is systematic can be improved.

If you practice and master this 3 step method and you dedicate yourself into learning and studying your every move like an art, I can practically guarantee that you will become a master at this and you can write your own ticket for how many clients you would like to have.

Let's take a look at this 3 step process and get right to it.

The 3 Step Sales Process

Master this process and your success will be unlimited

Let me introduce you to the sales process that has made a lot of money for a lot of personal trainers and gyms once they follow it. It has been the formula that has helped me sell several million dollars in gross sales in personal training. It is a simple formula that if you stay consistent and continuously work at it you will eventually become a very strong salesperson.

You will become more confident and excited in your business because you will know that you can create your own paycheck and you won't have to worry about if you will be able to pay the bills. Most personal trainers give up their training careers or keep it as a side job because they do not know how to sell.

If you master this sales process I guarantee that you will succeed. You will enjoy your job and everything that is has to offer much more and you will be able to maximize your potential. Now let's take a look at the sales process below.

The 3 Step Personal Training Sales Process

Step 1 - assessing the client's goals and building emotional rapport (most important step)
Step 2- putting the potential client through a workout (keep it dynamic, interesting, short, and educational)
Step 3- reviewing step 1 and 2 and closing the sale (if you do step 1 and 2 correctly this should be easy)

Step 1 (Assessing the clients goals and building emotional rapport)

The Goal of Step 1

The goal of Step 1 is to ask enough questions to reveal the emotional motivation of the client, educate the client on how to lift weights properly, eat healthily, and do the right amount of cardio based on their goals, and address any objections early on based off of the **FIT** principle.

Step 1 is all about building rapport, trust and excitement about personal training and changing their life.

Things to Look for in Step 1

You want to spend as much time as possible on the key emotional motivators of the client. What I mean by this is the second the client says anything that comes off as emotionally important to them, you want to stay on that subject for as long as possible and refer back to that goal through the entire presentation.

For example, if someone says they want to feel better about themselves, meaning they want more confidence, then you want to expand on that and not move on to the next question, but you want to ask

- How do they mean?
- What does confidence feel like?
- Do they currently feel confident now?
- How has being confident changed their life?

Then when you move on to Step 2 which we will talk about more shortly, you will also want, as you're exercising, to educate how the exercises you are doing will help them feel more confident in their life. After every set, you will want to explain how the exercises you are doing will build muscle, burn fat or build energy, and how those benefits will directly increase their confidence.

Another example is if the client wants to fit better in their clothes you will want to ask questions such as, Do you have a specific size of clothing you want to wear?, Where do you want to shop for your new wardrobe? , What areas of your body would you like to change so that you can fit better in your clothes?, and Why is it important for you to fit better into your clothes?

Now when you move to Step 2, the exercises that you will do, you will want to explain to them how, by doing these exercises, they will be able to eliminate their problem of not fitting into their clothes the way they want to.

If you see a client get emotional or cry during your presentation, do not overreact. Instead, relate with them as much as possible and show them that you, too, are a human being and understand what they are feeling. The best way, in my opinion, to show the client that you understand how they feel is to share stories of your past clients or stories of your life which we will talk about shortly.

How to figure out the client's goal

When you are in step one you must first understand what the client's goals are in order to help them. Selling personal training and sales in general is all about helping the person in front of you. If you do not start with that in mind you will not sell as much as you could because the client will be able to sense that and automatically resist.

The best ways to figure out the client's goals are to ask questions that pertain to the client such as

- What are your fitness goals?
- When were you in the best shape of your life?

- What areas of your body would you like to improve?
- How long have you been thinking about getting into the best shape of your life?

As you ask these questions the goal is to write down all of the answers and get as much information out of them for each question. A mistake many personal trainers make when asking these questions is just taking a surface answer.

A surface answer is an answer such as I want to get fit or I want to tone or bulk. These answers are not good enough to give the client the best opportunity to get help from you. Typically these answers are given because they are shy about sharing their deeper concerns and true wants.

For example a better answer to get would be, my fitness goals are to tone up my chest, back, reduce my body fat percentage, and I want to reach all of these goals because I want to be able to wear the clothes that I want with confidence without feeling self-conscious. Now that is a much better answer where you are able to direct the presentation with those focal points in mind.

The more in depth questions you ask of the client's goal the more likely that you are of presenting the personal training packages in a high value manner. Emotions are everything and below we will talk about how to touch them.

How to touch the emotions and figure out what is important to the client

Personal training sales is an emotional sale and if you do not discover what the emotional trigger is for the client on why they want to reach their specific goals then you will struggle to reach your potential in growing your business.

Emotions are what drives decisions and what drives all of us as human beings. I want you to think about the example of why someone buys a Mercedes Benz car. The purpose of a car is to get you to a specific destination which there are many cars that are much cheaper that can get the job done.

But that is not why Mercedes buyers buy Mercedes. They are buying the Mercedes for the emotion of feeling powerful, popular, superior, elegant, hardworking, etc. People buy things for what they will make them **FEEL** ultimately.

In personal training you must figure out why someone wants to get that set of nice abs or lose 40 pounds or whatever else their fitness goals are.

The most common reasons I hear are they want to increase their confidence, date more, fit better in their clothes, look better naked, be able to have more energy with their kids, improve their relationships, and improve their career performance.

In your presentation if you do not hear answers like these and you are only getting answers like I just want to get in shape then work on asking more questions and do not be afraid to dig deep.

Why It's Important to Get the Emotions of the Client

The reason why it's important to get the clients' emotions is because personal training is an emotional sale, it's not all logical. The best way to pull the emotions out is to make sure you're asking plenty of questions and using the word "why" often.

Some examples of questions are:

- Why do you want to lose weight?
- How long have you being thinking about losing weight, and how has it affected your life? Why?
- In what ways will getting to your fitness goals change your life? Why?
- How do you think you will feel when you achieve these goals? Why?
- In 12 months, what do you want to look like? Why?
- In 12 months, how do you want to feel? Why?

- How do you currently feel about your current fitness level? Why?
- How do you feel when you look in the mirror, and why?
- What are some trouble spots on your body that you would like to improve, and why?
- How do you think that getting into better shape will improve your relationships, life and career? Why?
- Are you looking to fit better in your clothes and feel better about what you wear? Why?

As you are getting the responses to this question you want to make sure that you are writing down all of their answers. This will make you seem more professional, engaged, and most important it allows you to take notes to know which direction you should take your sales presentation to.

The more information you get and the more questions you ask the better because it helps with connecting with the client and showing that you care and it will also get you more invested in the presentation.

You want to get yourself to the point to where you are feeling like you "have to" help. That you are so emotionally engaged with this person that if you were not to sell them you would feel like you let them down because you have the answers to their problems. This leads me to my next point which is the opposite of emotional selling but too many personal trainers try to sell this way and find out the hard way that people are not buying.

Logical Selling

Most personal trainers make the mistake of trying to sell personal training logically. For example, a personal trainer will try to sell how working out will increase muscle and help them lose weight. The trainers then go on and on and on with telling the client how many certifications they have, why they need to pay them to train them, why they have to eat a healthy diet etc. The problem with this is these are just logical reasons and logic is not enough to cause people to want to buy personal training.

Everyone knows what they should be doing because it is promoted advertised and drilled into their heads every day. So selling on logic is definitely important, but it is not where you want to spend most of your time on.

Another mistake personal trainer's make is they rely too much on logical tests such as just taking body fat, sit and reach test, and heart rate test, etc. These are all important in personal training somebody, but they alone will not sell somebody.

Everyone knows that they should exercise and eat right, but the problem is, the reason why they're not exercising and eating right is because they don't have enough emotional motivation to act. For example, wanting to lose 20 pounds is not enough to motivate someone to keep working out, but if you were to say, if you lose 20 pounds you will get a $10,000 a year raise at work, now that will motivate someone who is motivated by career progress or money, because there is an end result--a benefit for them.

Your job as a personal trainer is to sell benefits to the client. The logical part of selling should mostly consist of you explaining and educating them on the benefits THEY will be getting. People want to know what is in it for them so you might as well give it to them and spend most of your time talking about them.

You will notice a direct correlation with how much time is being spent talking about the client and your closing rate and income.

An Explanation of Features vs. Benefits

A feature is something that is part of the program or something you are selling. For example, if you're selling a car, a feature is, it has air conditioning. Now if you're selling personal training, a feature is that you're taking their body fat once a month.

Most trainers are selling features but they forget to sell the benefit. For example, personal trainers will sell how they will develop a workout program for their clients, or teach them how to eat correctly, or how they can give them varieties in their workouts, but they fail to explain the benefits of what those features will do for the client.

For example, you can say by developing a personalized workout program, the benefit the client will receive is they will be doing the correct workout for their personal results.

Benefits are what the client will receive and that is what they are truly interested in. Some examples of benefits are:
- increased self-esteem and confidence
- increased energy
- better relationships
- fit better in their clothes
- increased knowledge on how to exercise
- injury prevention and/or rehab
- better production at their work or career

I cannot stress enough how important it is to focus heavily on the benefits of what the client will get by training with you. When you think about how the client will benefit, your presentation and your attitude will shift from straight sales mode to help mode which will in turn impress the client and they will end up seeing the value and buying.

I have seen it over and over again where a personal trainer with a million certifications tries to sell a client and all that personal trainer does is sell their own ego and pride to the client and basically insulting the client in front of them because the client feels like they are being talked down to. That is what happens when the presentation is all about you when it should be about the client. So make sure your tone of voice and presentation are matched with who you are with.

Your Tone of Voice Matters

The key to tone of voice is that you do not want to be monotone. You want your tone of voice to go up and down as you show the benefits and ask questions. This will make sure the client is truly paying attention to what you are saying and it does cause an emotional response from the client as well. Pay very close attention to your tone of voice in your presentations because you may be saying all of the right things but how you are saying it is not conveying the message that you are trying to get across.

Your tone of voice can be the "make it or break it" and the responses you get in your presentation. As you're speaking and asking the questions, your tone of voice will want to fluctuate between high energy and empathy. It gives your presentation personality.

The reason why high energy and empathy in your presentation are important is because the client will mirror what you do. And that is one of the best ways to build leadership in your presentation is to create the energy in the environment.

The Mirroring Concept is how you lead the sales presentation

The mirror concept is, whatever body language the client has, you want to have congruent and similar body language. For example, if the client is leaning back, you want to lean back, so that the client feels comfortable and you are working at the pace of the client.

Think about why people dislike used car salesmen so much. The reason is the used car salesman is trying to pressure you or force you to do what he wants you do to, not what's best for you. The way he/she does this is by not paying attention to the details and body language of the customer and missing out on the key indicators of what the customer is feeling.

Subconsciously the customer can feel that and therefore puts a bad taste in the customer's mouth.

Some examples of bad mirroring would be if the used car salesman is leaning forward and giving off the perception that he wants you to choose the car that he wants to sell as opposed to sitting back and asking questions that are important to you, so he can show you the car that you want.

This is why mirroring is so important, because body language plays a big role in how we communicate.

Now I want you to work each day on mirroring a client

without coming off weird. You can practice it with your spouse, friends, whoever, to get the habit down. Next we will discuss how important it is to overcome objections early in step 1 and how to do so.

How to Overcome the Objections Early

The easiest way to overcome the objections early is to talk about them confidently and address them directly. By addressing the objections directly and early, it will cause the client to be more relaxed before you move on to Step 2.

The last thing you want to do when selling personal training is surprise the client at the end of the sale with the prices. You will lose trust from the client and they will resist buying from you because they will feel you were trying to hide something. Make sure as you are addressing the objections you calmly talk about that the program will cost money but there is a program that you can customize for them.

Resist the temptation to discuss the objection too long and try to close too early. The reason why you want to avoid trying to close too early is mostly for your benefit. What I mean is, if you try to close too early you may discourage yourself for the rest of the presentation because you may start to believe that they will not buy.

The correct way to handle objections early on is to address

the objections, provide a solution, show empathy, but not over-react to the objection. Your tone of voice and body language are key when hearing any form of resistance. Remember, you want to welcome the objection and show the client that you understand their concerns and you can find a solution to their worry.

Also, by not over-reacting to their objections, this shows that you are experienced and you are a professional, and know how to deal with clients just like them. Using stories is one of the best ways to help overcome objections early.

The Importance of Telling Stories and How to tell them

Telling stories of past clients or of your personal experiences are extremely powerful because it shows that you, too, understand how life can be and it creates a connection between you and the client.

Telling stories can be powerful also because no one wants to feel like they're the only one going through this problem and the story shows that a successful solution can be found.

Some examples of stories to share are the same stories that you may feel the client can relate to. Sometimes, if you have a feeling that the client might be embarrassed to admit a certain concern, such as feeling a lack of confidence, you can share a story first of when you felt a lack of confidence and how you overcame the problem.

By you telling a story of this first, shows that you are willing to be vulnerable and share a certain part of yourself to the client, but most importantly, it gives the client permission to now open up to you. That is what you call the Law of Reciprocation.

More stories you can tell that are powerful, are stories about you or other people losing weight, gaining muscle, going through adversity and overcoming it, or stories of how getting in better shape changed people's lives, particularly in their dating life or their relationships with their family. In my experience, these stories are what work the best in creating an emotional connection with the client. Don't be afraid to dig deep.

How to Overcome the Fear of Digging Too Deep

A common fear that personal trainers have is the fear of asking too personal of questions. This is a fear that you must get over as quickly as possible. If you do not dig deep and ask personal questions and you accept surface answers, such as, I just want to get in shape; you will have a much harder time signing up the client.

Remember the mirroring concept. If you feel uncomfortable, then the client will feel uncomfortable. What I recommend you do, if this is a problem area for you, is to find a friend or a partner to role play with and practice asking deeper questions and getting comfortable with it. This is the only way to get good at digging deep, practice.

Practicing and repetition was the only way that I got good at asking great questions. What I also recommend is, you write down 25 questions that you can practice and memorize so that when you are in a presentation, you have rehearsed so many times that the questions come naturally and you don't have to think about it.

The Importance of Role Play

Role playing is a drill that you must do with someone else whether you feel comfortable doing it or not. Most personal trainers feel embarrassed to role play, but don't let that be you, and let fear of embarrassment prevent you from being successful.

The best way to do role playing is to ask questions and practice hearing the responses and rehearsing your tone of voice and your reaction. You want the person you are role playing with to give you the hardest objections that you will face and not make it easy for you.

By having the person give you the hardest objections and keep saying them, this will force you to get better at your responses, so when your client is in front of you giving you objections, you have already practiced these objections for hours on end.

Role playing takes commitment and repetition every single day, and you also have to pay attention to the details, writing them down and understanding what is working for you and what is *not* working for you.

Do not be afraid to try new stories, responses, or questions that you asked during role play and use them in your actual presentation.

The only way to get good at communicating and responding to objections is to pay very close attention and break down even the minutest detail of your interaction.

For example, by saying what do you mean? As opposed to how do you mean? Can make a difference on how someone responds to you. It can be the difference between building a connection with the client and offending the client. This is why role playing is so important.

The Education of Weight Training, Nutrition and Cardio

The key when you're educating the client (in step 1) about these topics are you want to explain in regular English or regular language how to do each of the steps correctly.

The key points in the education of weight training is you want to explain the importance of variety in their workout, and changing their workout routines often, and then explain to them how this will help them to avoid hitting a plateau.

When you're talking about weight training, you do want to show your knowledge about drop sets, supersets, straight sets and reps and all of the logistics of training. Also, it's important to talk about periodization and other weight training concepts, but you do not want to overwhelm them with too many big terms or concepts or you will scare them away.

Educating the client on nutrition, the key points you want to explain are macronutrients (protein, carbs and fat), nutrient timing, eating often, and meal planning etc. You do not want to break down too much information and bore the client to death about how everything works. Just explain how you can help organize the nutrition and save them time.

When educating about cardio, you want to explain the fundamentals of running, biking, cycling, and any other form of cardio exercise and how it will help them achieve their goals. Use the same principles you used in nutrition education which is show them how you will help organize and save their time in their workouts.

The education of weights, cardio, and nutrition part of step 1 should be brief and concise and should clearly demonstrate the benefits of having an organized program personalized for the client.

This is not a time to recite the entire NASM or ACE book. This will kill your sales more than anything else if you over-educate them in Step 1.

Preparing for Step 2 (The Workout)

When preparing for Step 2 (The Workout), you will want to make sure that you are bringing up that you will be giving them a sample workout to see how it will be to work with a personal trainer and then, if they would like a personal trainer, it will cost money.

This is extremely important to bring up before you go into the workout so that it does not surprise the client that the training comes for free. You want to prepare the client because that shows respect and it will also lower buyer's resistance.

The last thing you want to do is build rapport and get the client excited for personal training and then surprise them with a hidden cost or fee. This is a step that most personal trainers skip and then wonder why they cannot seem to sell their clients.

So, an example phrase that you would want to use before going into Step 2, "Today I am going to show you what it's like to work with a personal trainer and show you what your workouts should look and feel like. If personal training is something that you would like to purchase at the end, I will show you the prices for our programs and you can choose whatever program that you would like. If not, no big deal. I am still here to help you."

Step 2: The Workout

Create a Standardized Workout

You must create a standardized workout that can be changed based on the client's goals, fitness levels and injuries. I typically recommend you choose five to seven different exercises for your workout.

The reason why you want to create a standardized workout especially when you're beginning to learn this sales approach is that you will want to be able to rehearse the same process over and over again so you can find ways to improve it easier.

The workout's purpose is to educate and demonstrate the value of having someone help the client in their workout. During the standardized workout, the purpose is to ask questions while the client is performing the exercises then show how the exercises done your way will help the client achieve their goals.

An example of a standardized workout would be:

- a squat
- a pushup or bench exercise for chest
- a pull or row exercise for back
- a lunge or a step up for legs
- some sort of core or abdominal exercise

How to Adjust the Standardized Workout

Most personal trainers are afraid to standardize a workout because they fear that they are being too generic, but what most personal trainers find is, by rehearsing and performing the standardized workout over and over again, it gives them a chance to memorize a system that allows them to be creative.

What I mean by this is, if you've memorized the system and you've done so many repetitions of it, you will no longer have to think about what you're going to do with the client, therefore allowing you to be more creative in what you say and do in your workouts.

Most personal trainers get hung up on not knowing what workouts they should do with the client in the free orientation or session. That causes them to randomly create a workout routine that is not as powerful and also causes the personal trainer anxiety, which causes them to not be able to sell the client because they are thinking of too many things at once.

The way you adjust the standardized workout will be based on the client's abilities. For example, if a client is older and has had problems with the lower half of their body, you can do the squat but modify it to maybe a bodyweight squat or ball squat.

On the flipside, if you have an advanced client, then you can do exercises such as a bosu ball squat or you can use more advanced techniques, such as a drop set. As you can see, the standardized workout is just a template to use. So be creative and focus mostly on what you will say and when you will say it in your workouts.

Questions to Ask During the Workout

As you're doing the workout, in between sets be sure to ask questions that show the client the value of what you are doing. For example, after you complete a set, you should be asking questions such as:

- Did you feel the difference when I corrected your technique?
- Do you notice how the shortening up of rest between sets gives you a better workout?
- Can you see how doing workouts like these will help you lose weight, gain muscle, drop body fat, increase endurance, etc.?
- Do you see how, by having a plan, your workouts are better, because you are not thinking about what you will do next?

Those are just some sample questions that I recommend you use during the workout to show the value of a personal trainer and have the client sell themselves. Asking questions during the workout is extremely important in selling and engaging with the client.

I suggest you come up with 15 to 20 of your own questions that you rehearse and memorize every day to use during the workouts. Make sure you write these down on paper so that you do not forget, and make these questions real.

How Many Sets Should You Do in This Workout?

I personally think you should not do any more than two sets per exercise in order to prevent boredom. The way you dictate how many sets, whether that be one or two, will be based on the client's ability and attention span.

This is where you need to use your intuition to read how engaged the client is in the workout.

Some signs to look for as far as engagement is concerned are, how they're breathing, how many questions they're asking, and what their motivation level appears to be.

If you see signs of good eye contact, excitement, and a very high level of interest on what you're teaching them, these are called buying signals. Make sure that when the client shows you buying signals you are communicating that personal training is right for them and reconfirm what they are saying to keep the sales momentum going.

Machines vs. Free Weights and Body Weight in Step 2

In order to show the most value in having a personal trainer, you will want to do exercises and movements that the client normally does not do on their own. What I mean is, typically clients can figure out how to use gym machines and equipment.

If you show them machines as part of your presentation, it will give the client the perception that they can do it on their own, and that they do not need you as a personal trainer.

A big mistake personal trainers make when selling clients is, they choose to do machines over free weights, because it appears to be safer and less work. In actuality, this will significantly decrease the engagement of the client and lower your chances of selling the client.

In my experience, showing clients exercises using their own body weight or free weights is the best way to show the value of personal training. The reason this is the best way to show value is that the movements are most likely foreign to the client and allows you more opportunity to correct and engage with the client.

There are exceptions to using machines as part of your presentation. What I recommend is using cables or suspension training as the machines of choice to demonstrate the value of personal training. I would first stick with free weight and body weight exercises until you become very skilled at selling personal training.

The Pace of the Workout

The pace of the workout should be geared toward the client in front of you, so if you have a younger, more athletic client that you are trying to sell, the speed of your workout should be relatively quick. It should be high-energy, motivating, and "almost infomercial-like."

If you have an older client with injuries, then your workout should be mostly educational and slower. After every set, you should explain to the client why you are doing the exercise and how it will benefit them.

The pace of the workout should be well-balanced with education and energy. You want to be careful not to do too much of one or the other. Pay very close attention to your energy prior to doing the workout. For example, if you are going to need high energy for the presentation, you should have a routine that you follow to prepare yourself.

Do as much research as possible on the client you will be presenting to, so you can prepare yourself accordingly. Preparation is everything when it comes to the workout. Be sure to get yourself in the correct state.

How to Lead the Workout

It's very important that you have a structured workout so that you have a direction to lead the client to. You will want to demonstrate leadership qualities as a trainer by consistently telling the client what to do next. For example, you'll want to tell them:

- to go get a drink of water
- to move here or there
- how many more reps they should do
- how much longer they'll be resting
- to contract their muscles
- to notice how it feels

The reason why you want to use these in the workout, is to train the client to get used to taking direction in the personal training session. This is often a reason why a client buys. They do not want to have to think about what to do next, therefore, they'll hire you.

How to Smoothly Transition from the Workout to the Close

At the end of the workout session, most personal trainers start to feel very high anxiety about transitioning to asking for the sale, therefore, this is an extremely important subject to cover.

The best way to transition from the workout to the close is to make sure you are controlling your emotions and slowing everything down in your head.

The client will mirror what you are doing so if you seem nervous they will feel nervous. The key here is to manage yourself and understand it is all in your head. Ask plenty of yes questions at this stage to make sure they are getting in the mode of saying yes and getting emotionally involved in what you are saying.

You want to have a good balance of high energy and excitement while being relaxed to demonstrate that you have sold personal training before and this is no big deal to you. You want to have the mentality of everyone that meets with you buys from you.

Take the lead and be sure that you ask a buying question at the end of every rebuttal statement you make. A few examples are

- Do you want to use an American express, Visa, etc?
- So would you like to do the 2 or the 3 times per week program?
- Do you prefer a male or female trainer?

How to create urgency

Now the next step is to get the client to want to buy from you today. This is a skill that you must learn if you are going to sell a lot of personal training. In order for someone to feel a sense of urgency to buy something you have to apply skillful pressure.

A good way to do that is when you ask them to buy you don't say anything until they speak first. Another technique you can use to create urgency is to talk about the limited schedule that you have and how fast it is getting booked so if they are serious about training and want to get going with you then they will want to sign up now to lock their spot in.

Another way to create urgency is to use tie downs about how long they have been thinking about getting into shape. An example would be "it has been 5 years since you were in the best shape of your life, so you have been thinking about getting back into shape for about 5 years right? It seems like you are ready to change so let's get you going"

Another way to create urgency is to bring it up early in step 1 of your sales process saying things such as what has been holding you back from reaching the goals that you want and why have they been holding you back? And then follow up with a question such as are you ready and committed to start getting the results you want now?

Key point here is if you want to create urgency the best way is to combine high emotion with high value of training. You want them to feel the emotion of happy and excited about what is possible for them in the future and have them picture in their head while building the massive amount of value in having a personal trainer that motivates them and does almost all of the work for them by giving them the best workout regimens out there.

If you can get the client to be in a highly emotional state AND show them the value of training you will be able to close more people easier with minimal objections. You will know you are doing it right when the close takes 5 minutes or less for them to make a decision.

Selling is about leadership and guidance and the better you are at doing those two things the more sales you will make.

Step 3 (Recap and Close)

The FIT System a.k.a. the objections

The FIT system stands for **F**inancial, **I** need to think about it or procrastinate, and **T**ime.

These are the three most common objections that you will face when selling personal training. Your goal is to address and overcome these objections **before** Step 2 of the process.

The financial objections typically mean that you did not show enough value for what you are charging for personal training. For example, during the recession, the company Apple had one of the most successful years. The reason is even though people felt cash-stressed, the value of purchasing an IPhone or IPad was great enough to buy.

Some of the best ways to overcome the financial objections are to ask questions that isolate the problem. One of my personal favorite questions to ask when I get objections is…. How do you mean?

The purpose of the question is to isolate exactly what the client means such as is the down-payment the issue or is it the monthly investment?

Logically you cannot overcome the financial objection by telling them to cut out going to the movies or cutting out fast food, because those are not emotional motivations. What I mean is, that seems to the client like a negative motivation because no one likes to be told what they cannot do. Instead of logically overcoming the financial objections, you need to demonstrate the value to justify the financial commitment. Use as much emotion as possible to overcome the financial objections.

I need to think about or procrastinate objection means that you have not demonstrated the value of buying personal training right now. This typically means that you did not create enough urgency and value by explaining to them the reasons why they need to get started now. Some ways to create urgency is by asking questions such as, how long have been wanting to reach your fitness goals? Another question you can ask is when was the last time you were in the best shape of your life?

I want you to have the client verbally paint the picture answering the question, "If you started a plan to reach your goals 12 months ago, where would you be today? Follow up with the question, where do you want to be 12 months from now, and have the client paint that picture.

Oftentimes you will get this objection if you are doing very easy workouts, too many machine workouts, or you did not create a strong enough emotional reaction in step 1. If you get this, focus on doing step 1 better and creating more urgency.

When you get the **time objection**, you typically want to respond by asking, how do you mean? And have the client isolate what they mean. For example, the time objection can actually mean that they think they have to keep a schedule, or the fear if they don't schedule the sessions they will lose the sessions.

The time objection, like the rest of the objections, are usually solvable and it's a misunderstanding from the client's perspective. That is why it is extremely important to isolate the objection so you are overcoming the true objection.

For the most part, every other objection, including the spouse objection, fall under the FIT system. For example, if a husband or wife says they need to speak with their spouse before they sign up, they typically have an objection of finances, I need to procrastinate, time. You just have isolate and discover what the true objection is.

Isolating the Objection

What you have to focus on when someone resists buying a personal training program is to truly figure out the main concern that is holding them back from getting started today. Sometimes you have to isolate and re-isolate several times before you get to the true objection. Sometimes people are afraid to tell you the true objection for fear of upsetting you or they are embarrassed.

Some of the best ways to isolate the objection is to ask how do you mean? And then re-state the objection back to the client so you can clarify if that's the true objection. For example, if the client gives you the money objection and says I can't afford it, then you'll ask how do you mean and then the client may say back to you, I can't afford to pay all of this money up front. Now you have discovered the true objection is the down-payment or what they have to pay today. So, now you have an objection to work with and overcome.

A side note on objections, you objections in your presentation. Most trainers think objections are bad, but the reason why objections are good is because they usually show a sign of interest, because if a client doesn't have any objections and says nothing, then you have nothing to work with, so welcome objections.

Isolating the objection may be one of the most important things to get really good at because you can use it at any point of the sale to clearly communicate the necessary information to overcome any hesitation.

The reason why you really want to isolate the true objection is because you want to narrow it down to one objection. Trying to overcome five objections at the end of the sale such as I can't afford this, I need to speak to my wife, and I don't know if I have time, is extremely difficult to overcome.

Controlling your emotions during the close

During the close most personal trainers allow themselves to show too much emotion and it is usually the type of emotion that is negative which is not good because the client can feel that. The more the client can feel the negative emotion the more they are hesitant to buy from you.

The best way to control your emotions at the close is to make sure you are detaching yourself from the outcome and you are breathing and giving yourself positive feedback in your head while asking them to buy the package. This does take some practice because in the beginning when you are first starting to sell, you will be nervous.

The faster you learn how to manage these emotions the faster you will build up your client base and the happier and more successful you will be. It is not uncommon to get high anxiety at this point of the sales process because the client is scared to get "closed" and you are scared that you will not get "paid".

This is the point of the sale where thinking positively is crucial because if you are thinking positively and you go into the sale thinking that good things will happen then good things will happen.

My personal philosophy is every presentation is a sale for me. I am selling them on the benefits and if they don't buy from me today they will eventually buy or sell their friends on the training because I demonstrated the value.

When you know you are selling correctly

You will know when you are selling correctly when you are making the client feel so comfortable that they feel they can confide in you and you will not judge them or give them a negative reaction. The client will basically feel like they are the one in control and if they tell you no they don't have to avoid you or have that awkward feeling of no longer being able to communicate with you because they said no.

The best way to do this is to make sure you are not hard closing the client by making them feel like if they don't buy right now you are going to freak out or have a negative reaction. Showing them empathy on what their concerns are and making a point to show them that you are trying to find solution to their concern goes a long way.

Keep the phrase in your mind "sell to help".

Section 2-
Marketing

"You can't sell to
an empty chair"

Marketing personal training is something that if you master you can control your own income, schedule, and growth. This specific business skill will take you from not having a plan on how to get your next client to knowing exactly step by step and systematically how to get clients into your sales funnel so you can start changing their lives.

You most likely got involved in personal training because you want to help people change their lives and personal training seemed like a good career to do that. The problem with the personal training certification process is they do not teach in depth on how to actually GET clients.

Once you graduate or get certified you are kind of left on your own to figure out how to start making money. As personal trainers we all want to be able to make a living and have the CHOICE to make personal training a side job or a career.

In this section I will teach you the EXACT marketing strategies that I have used to sell millions of dollars' worth of personal training packages. I will break down the different ways to generate leads so you can funnel them into the 3 step sales process.

We will cover phone calls, email blasts, floor pulls, social media, direct mail, magazine contributing etc. There are many different techniques and strategies that you can use in order to build up your client base and of course your income.

So now we are going to get right into it. Make sure to read and re read this section as it will guaranteed make you money and the more you perfect these strategies and build on them the more confidence you will have when it comes to marketing yourself and your packages.

Where to start …. The Who

The first thing you want to do when you are starting or strategizing on how you will build up your client base is to write down on a piece of paper who you are trying to sell to or attract. This is a step that if you don't start with it you will be doing a lot of busy work and you can't systematize your efforts.

There are a few questions that you want to ask and write down and save and they are

- What is the age range you are trying to attract? (example: 25-35 years old)

- Are you trying to attract women or men?

- How much income does your potential client make?

- Where/what does your potential client work or do all day?

- What are the biggest fears of your potential clients?

- What problems do you solve for your potential clients?

- What do your potential clients read and watch?

- What will be your unique selling proposition? (example: expert at training stay at home moms)

- What forms of communication will you use to speak to your potential clients? (example: email)

- What are the emotional triggers of your potential clients? (fear, pride, power, etc)

DO NOT SKIP THIS EXERCISE. This is the basis of your business right here. Personal training is a business so make sure you are treating it as such.

The more focused and clear about who you are trying to sell the more successful your efforts will be. The biggest mistake personal trainers make when they are trying to increase their clients is they are trying to speak to everybody and they don't have a focused message.

If you try to sell everybody you will end up selling nobody because your message will be too diluted and plain and it won't speak to anyone powerfully enough therefore you won't attract clients.

The goal in marketing is to attract clients to want to come to you and have them tell their friends who also fit your customer profile.

Do not be afraid to niche down your message because your message may still attract people who don't fit your exact demographic but they are attracted to your message.

Keep this sheet of paper that you answered the questions on and have that be your guide to everything that you do when you are building your client base. Those answers should be very helpful to crafting your message.

Your Message to your Market

Now that you know exactly who you are trying to sell to, the next thing you must do is create your emotionally charged message that matches and speaks to your particular group.

How NOT to have your message match your market is to create a plain message that doesn't resonate with your group. For example if you are selling to 25-35 year old stay at home mom and your marketing message is you do sport specific training and powerlifting then that is not going to attract them to contact you.

But, if your message to the 25-35 year old stay at home mom is something like "I help stay at home moms get there pre baby body back" then that will at least get their attention and they will know that you are potentially the trainer for them!

There are many different messages that make a difference in who you attract. Now, what you want to think about in your strategy is how you can create the image that is necessary complimented with the right words and communication strategy to get the attention of the market you want.

So using the 25-35 year old stay at home mom as our example, you would want to have pictures of what your potential client most likely wants to look like on your marketing material.

Now be very aware of what pictures you choose to use for your advertisements because if you choose a picture of a lady who looks too perfect and like she has never had a baby before it will turn off the potential client.

The picture has to be of someone who is considered to be just like them. The closer the picture looks like the potential client or what is believed as "possible" the stronger it is.

Now your actual wording of the message must be interesting and also spark a reaction by bringing out the problems your potential client is most likely having and/or feeling and how you can solve those feelings and problems fast.

So earlier you wrote down your potential client profile. What you are going to do next is take the information that you wrote down and then craft a message. When you craft the message you want to think that you are only talking to one individual.

The more it feels like you are talking just to them individually, the more powerful the message. If it feels like it is just a mass message the potential client will most likely not be interested in what you have to say.

The <u>most powerful message</u> that you can create to spark their attention is a story of someone else who looks, feels, struggled, and overcame the same problems that your potential client has.

The reason this works so well is it speaks directly to the emotions of your potential client and hits their emotional triggers. The story allows the client to put themselves in the shoes of the storyteller and realize that they too have had these same issues.

It essentially gives the potential client hope that they can get help, that there is a solution and the potential client will associate the story with your service. That is powerful.

Action steps

1. Complete your customer profile and post it on your wall, fridge, and anywhere else that you will see it so it is a reminder of who you are talking to.

2. Create a clear marketing message to your customer profile that talks about their fears and problems and how you can solve them

3. Compile 3-4 emotionally charged stories that will resonate with your customer profile so you can repurpose them. (example email, video interview, magazine article, etc)

Distribution of Your Message

Once you know who you are trying to target and you craft the message that you want to say to them the next step you are going to want to do is figure out how you will get the message out.

There are many different methods and strategies that you can use in order to get the sales to come through the door but I am going to mainly discuss the ones that have worked for me.

The very first thing you will want to do is if you are currently working out of a gym and you have an arrangement with the gym where you are paying them rent then you will want to start with this tip I am about to give you.

You will want to ask the gym if you can get access to the email list and mailing list of the current members of the gym. As many famous marketers have said before, the money is in the list. The client list is the most valuable asset you can have in my opinion because if you have a list you can always create something for them to buy.

Now when you get their email list what you will want to do next is get all of their emails in a spreadsheet and then move them into an email software where you can manage the names and track open rates, delivery rates, etc

The software that I like to use is called mail chimp but there are others out there such as constant contact and Aweber. The key is to find a software that you feel comfortable using and learn the ins and outs of it. It will normally cost you less than $50 a month for this service. Trust me the investment in this is well worth your money.

After you upload your list the next thing you will want to do is to start creating your next email campaign which will be a campaign where you send an invite to the mailing list introducing yourself and the offer you would like to give them.

Now it is very important that you don't come off as spammy or as a pest so when you send your email make sure to tell them why you are emailing them, how you can help them, and offer them a free fitness assessment where you will sit down with them and go over their goals and help them come up with a structured plan based off of their goals.

Also make sure they know very clearly they can opt out of this email list if they want to because you want to have a clean list of people who want to actually hear from you as opposed to people who will be upset that you are emailing them.

The next step is to at least twice a week send them something of value that they can use immediately in the gym and at the end of every piece of content always have a call to action to schedule their free fitness assessment with you.

This is the way to generate a lot of appointments fast and it is very efficient as you don't have to go door to door to get their attention.

Some key points when you are emailing the client list to schedule an appointment are

- Make sure you are consistent (at least 1 email per week)

- Give away your best content for free (this builds trust)

- Focus on creating compelling headlines (so people actually open your emails)

- Test often to see which campaigns work the best (so you can use them in the future)

The next technique you will want to use to start scheduling appointments is the customer calling list. You will want to take the calling list of the members of the gym and start offering them a complimentary fitness assessment.

Now, when you are making these phone calls you don't want to schedule dead appointments. What I mean by dead appointments is if you are only offering a free session and then setting up a time where they come to meet you but you are not finding out what their goals are then you are going to notice that none of your appointments that you schedule will show up.

The goal when making the phone call with each one of the members is to find out what their specific goals are and gather as much information as you can from them over the phone so you can customize their fitness assessment.

By getting more information over the phone and spending at least 3-5 minutes on the phone talking with them, they will see more value in coming in to your appointment and they will also trust you more because you are asking them questions that other people don't ask them.

The types of questions that you want to ask them over the phone are questions that pertain to what their fitness goals are, how long have they been trying to achieve those goals, what struggles and obstacles have they ran into, etc.

The goal is to dig as deep as you can on these questions getting answers such as I have been trying to lose this weight for five years, I have low self-confidence and I want to change, I want to fit back into my clothes again but I don't know what to do etc

Once you schedule the appointment tell them exactly what action step you want them to do and that you will be calling to confirm their appointment on the day of or day before. The key to taking leadership on this process is if you tell them what to do they will feel like you are a professional and you know exactly what you are doing.

Perception is everything so make your first impression count by doing the things that are going to help them feel more comfortable and trust you more.

Typically you want to make phone calls every day if you are trying to quickly build up your clients and increase your income. This is also an area where you want to track how many phone calls you are making and when the best times to call people are.

If you are not having success calling people at a certain time then make sure to call them at a different time because it could just be the time of the day that you are calling that is causing you not to get appointments.

A key note on phone calls, one of the best things to do if you are not getting people to answer is to send them a quick text saying who you are and why you are calling them and then have a call to action. Now you want to be sensitive when you are texting people because you also don't want them to feel too pushed so don't apply too much pressure via text because that will turn the client off.

When you shoot them a text the goal is to ask them for permission for when a good time would be to call them for a "short call" to discuss scheduling an appointment with you. The goal of every interaction when you make your first contact is to establish trust and schedule free fitness assessments so you have clients to sell to.

The next technique you will use to schedule appointments is the "floor pull or floor approach". The best way to approach this is you want to make an introduction to the people who are working out and letting them know that you are here to help and if they have any questions they can always reach out to you. You want to make sure you are not coming off intimidating or unapproachable because if you do then you will have a hard time having conversations that can turn into appointments.

With the floor pull approach you want to find ways to lead the conversation into what the client's specific goals are and then you want to give them a few quick tips that will be helpful for them to use right away and then you want to go into offering them a free fitness assessment.

The same rule applies to this technique just like every other technique which is to make sure you are not setting dead appointments and you are digging deep. The longer you spend on communicating with the client in front of you when it comes to their goals and what they want to achieve the more likely that person will show up to your appointment.

The next technique you will want to use is you will want to have a strong presence on social media so you can keep your name and services in the top of your clients' minds so they know who to go to with fitness questions.

Social media is a great way to establish trust within your community and also it is a way to brand yourself as the fitness guy/girl. Just like email if you are posting consistently and you are posting content that is useful then you will be the person the client thinks of first when they think about fitness questions that they have.

The value in social media is it is a place where you can test out what people respond to and what they don't respond to as well. It is a great testing platform to gauge interest levels in different programs, offerings, specials, etc.

When you choose social media channels make sure you are choosing two to three of the most important social media channels that your customers are on. You don't have to be on EVERY social media channel because some of those channels may not make sense for who you are targeting.

A good example, is if you are marketing to males who want to become bigger and more muscular then Pinterest is probably not going to be the best channel for you to be on because Pinterest's demographic is mostly women.

You may also want to explore doing social media promoted posts and ads. Now these do cost money but it can be money well spent if you know what you are doing and you are clear on who you are targeting and what your message will say.

Social media is all about putting the clients through a gradual funnel so they are slowly getting to know you better and you aren't just shouting BUY MY STUFF on your channel.

The type of social media content that has been successful for me is content that drives them to a webpage that offers them more information that the clients can use. An example would be offering a free e book about some subject that your target market is interested in.

Another piece of social media content that has been very useful for me is the use of video trailers to promote personal training. The videos are created to build an emotional connection and excitement towards working out and bettering themselves.

This does not have to be expensive to create but it does have to have some creativity and thought put into it so people can relate to what you are showing them.

The next technique you want to use is the direct mailer strategy where you create a postcard that fits all the criteria of your customer profile and then you want it to be sent to their mailing addresses.

Now this technique can be very powerful if you do the postcard correctly and you have a compelling message with a strong offer to come in and see you.

The goal with this direct mail piece is to drive a response to come in for their free fitness assessment but this also is a branding tool so they will know who you are and start to see the images of what you do. Sometimes it does take quite a few interactions before anyone buys.

The way to speed up the sales cycle is for the clients to see you across multiple different medias because that will give what is called by many marketers as the "surround sound effect". What this means is everywhere that the client goes they are seeing and hearing about you.

This gives the perception that you are an expert in the marketplace and it also gives you social proof that if you are doing all of these methods you must be good. Direct mail is just like email and social media which consistency is key.

The more consistent you are the better results you will get in your marketing mix.

Being a contributor to a magazine, trade association, or anything that is related to personal training is a great way to establish yourself as an expert. If you are being seen in a magazine you will automatically have credibility that you know what you are talking about.

Once you have this credibility your opinion will have a much more powerful effect. This helps to pre sell someone before they ever come into one of your presentations or sessions.

In the magazine articles you typically want to choose magazines that are targeting the kind of clients that you want. So if you are trying to attract females who are family oriented make sure you are picking a magazine that reflects that.

The next thing you would want to do after that is you would write an article on a problem that most of your target market faces when they are trying to get into shape. This is a good time to try and overcome their objection in the article. For example, if you get a lot of money objections then in the article you would want to discuss how getting in shape can actually save them money and even better, make them more money.

Magazine articles are really helpful to expand your exposure and if you do that in addition to the marketing methods that we have talked about above it makes all of your marketing that much more effective.

Seminars/public speaking are a way to merge a sales presentation and writing an article and putting it on steroids. The reason this is such a powerful way to get leads is it shows you that you are the expert and you are giving value and it also allows the audience to get to know you and trust you more.

Seminars will help you speed up the sales cycle because instead of having to send a bunch of direct mail or emails or anything else for that matter they get a chance to hear you speak and see how you communicate for 30 minutes to an hour.

This could be equivalent to writing 20 or more articles as far as building trust and rapport is concerned. When choosing a topic to discuss choose topics that are pain points for your clients. These could be things such as how to fit back into their clothes or being able to get a new wardrobe.

Those would be the benefit you would be selling and the topic that you would discuss is how to maximize their nutrition to get the fastest and longest lasting results possible.

Advertising such as Tv, billboard, and movie theatres can be great ways to expose your brand and what you are trying to offer.

There are pros and cons to doing advertising in this way. The pros of doing advertising this way is you are automatically seen as a legitimate "big business" when you advertise, the cons to advertising this way is it is very expensive to use these kinds of media.

The other thing you will want to pay close attention to is how you design your advertising and making sure it has a direct response mechanism in it so you can track how well your advertising is doing.

 I would suggest you create a separate web page that only the people who see this specific advertisement go to and use a software like google analytics to track how many visitors you are getting and what your conversion rate is.

How to put all of these techniques together so you can start seeing results immediately!

With all of the ideas that I have given you above I want you to choose 3-5 different Medias that you will use to get the message out to your market.

Think this through before you just choose any random media so you are making sure you are getting in front of the people who really are your potential future clients.

Once you choose the media types I want you to create specific goals so you know if you are succeeding or not. For example, you would say my goal for my marketing campaign is to get 10 new leads per week using x, y, and z methods.

This way you can tweak what you are doing if necessary or really amplify what you are doing to get the results you want. The name of the game is to get as many qualified leads that you possibly can to get in front of you so you can offer your services.

After you set your goal you will then want to come up with a structured process of how you want to roll out your plan so all of your campaigns go together and are promoting the special offer.

The more sequenced and congruent the marketing campaigns are with each other the more successful your campaigns will be, guaranteed. When people see something over and over again they start to take it as safe and legitimate.

My Final Thoughts

Personal training can be a lucrative career and one of my goals is to change the perception that personal training is just a profession for people who don't want to have a real job or that personal training is just a side job and/or a stepping stone for another career. I want to be able to offer the best advice possible in order to get personal trainers to buy into the fact that they can make as much money as they want AND change people's lives.

You can do both, you don't have to choose just making money or just changing people's lives. It is possible to have it all if you are willing to work at your craft every day. Spend as much of your time as possible perfecting your sales and marketing process and how you communicate.

Great selling is just a form of high level communication and getting good at selling personal training will not only get you more clients it will help you in other areas of your life.

If you are serious about growing your personal training business then you will want to master how to market and sell personal training. This will take you and your business to the next level because it provides leverage.

Consistency and tracking are the key when you are selling and marketing and always remember that whatever gets measured gets improved. Hold yourself accountable and have fun while you are on the journey because it will be exciting when you start to see the sales coming in.

I hope you enjoyed this book and I recommend that you review it over and over again to get better at you what you are doing. Good luck in your career and make sure to visit my website www.thefiture.co for more education and products to help you take your personal training career to the next level.

Made in United States
North Haven, CT
28 October 2022

26025015R00039